# Dengue Pandemic

## Tracking the Most Rapidly Spreading Mosquito-Borne Disease

**Isabella White**

# Contents

# Foreword

As an epidemiologist who has spent over two decades studying arboviruses and the burden of mosquito-borne diseases, I have witnessed firsthand the alarming emergence and expansion of dengue across the globe. When I began my career in the 1990s, dengue was considered a tropical disease of relatively minor importance. Today, it is the fastest-spreading vector-borne viral disease in the world, with over half of the world's population at risk.

In this seminal new book, Dr. Isabella White provides a comprehensive and sobering look at the unfolding dengue pandemic. With insightful analysis and synthesis of the latest research, she tracks the forces driving the rapid dissemination of this dreaded disease. Unchecked urbanization, a lack of efficient mosquito control, the effects of climate change, international travel and trade, and the peculiarities of mosquito biology and dengue epidemiology that make containment so challenging all contribute to the dengue virus's global spread. As Dr. White makes clear, this is a complex global crisis with no simple solutions.

Providing historical context, up-to-date maps and data, and perspectives from the front lines, this book highlights the immense challenges we face in halting dengue's expansion.

From detailed chapters on dengue virology, Aedes mosquito ecology, surveillance systems, and vaccine research, Dr. White constructs a comprehensive picture of the dengue pandemic. While obstacles abound, the book ends with a roadmap and cautious optimism about future progress in dengue mitigation if we can muster the will and resources.

As we confront the sobering realities of an intensifying dengue pandemic, this book is an indispensable resource for public health professionals, infectious disease researchers, policymakers, and anyone seeking to understand what can be done to counter this growing threat. We ignore the dengue crisis only at great peril to public health worldwide.

**Laurel Hernandez, PhD**

*Professor of Epidemiology, School of Public Health*

# Introduction

Dengue fever, once considered a sporadic tropical disease, has now escalated into a major global health crisis. The dengue pandemic we are witnessing today threatens more than half the world's population and imposes immense health, economic, and social burdens. Over the last 50 years, dengue has undergone explosive expansion worldwide, with epidemics accelerating in frequency and magnitude.

Globally, the number of dengue cases reported to the World Health Organization increased eightfold from the 1960s to the 2010s. No longer confined to the tropics, dengue continues to extend its reach into sub-tropical and even temperate regions.

So why has this once obscure virus that was only identified in 1943 become the most rapidly spreading mosquito-borne disease? What perfect storm of factors has driven the global emergence of dengue on such a massive scale? In this book, I seek to answer these questions and unpack the complexities of the escalating dengue pandemic.

By synthesizing historical data, epidemiological research, virological and entomological studies, and on-the-ground perspectives, I aim to provide a comprehensive look at where dengue came from, how it spreads, and why controlling it has proven so challenging.

From the origins of dengue's four distinct serotypes to the intricacies of Aedes mosquito behavior that facilitate viral transmission, this book explores dengue from all angles. Gaps in our understanding of dengue pathogenesis, lack of effective therapies, challenges in developing a broadly protective vaccine, difficulties sustaining vector control, and limitations of surveillance systems are all examined. These weaknesses in dengue prevention and control are highlighted as factors enabling this virus to exploit our hypermobile, urbanized world.

As dengue cases continue to reach new record highs worldwide, there is urgency to rein in this runaway pandemic. This book provides a blueprint for the innovative strategies and multifaceted efforts needed at local and global levels to mitigate the immense threat posed by the dengue virus and Aedes mosquitoes.

With emerging tools and technologies, political will, targeted funding, and evidence-based policies, we can change the trajectory of the dengue pandemic. But, as readers will learn, we have no time to waste.

**Dr. Isabella White**

# Chapter 1

# Understanding Dengue Fever

## What is Dengue Fever?

The dengue virus, which causes dengue fever, spreads to people when infected mosquitoes, primarily the Aedes aegypti mosquito, bite a person. It is one of the most rapidly spreading mosquito-borne diseases in the world, affecting millions of people annually. The disease is prevalent in tropical and subtropical regions, particularly in urban and semi-urban areas.

The dengue virus belongs to the Flaviviridae family and has four distinct serotypes: DEN-1, DEN-2, DEN-3, and DEN-4. Each serotype can cause dengue fever, and infection with one serotype does not provide immunity against the others. Subsequent infections with different serotypes can lead to more severe forms of the disease, such as dengue hemorrhagic fever (DHF) and dengue shock syndrome (DSS).

The symptoms of dengue fever typically appear 4–7 days after the mosquito bite and can last for up to 10 days. The most common symptoms include high fever, severe headache, joint and muscle pain, rash, and mild bleeding from the nose or gums. In some cases, dengue fever can progress to DHF or DSS, which are characterized by severe bleeding, organ damage, and a drop in blood pressure. These severe forms of dengue fever can be life-threatening if not promptly diagnosed and treated.

Dengue fever is primarily transmitted through the bite of infected female Aedes mosquitoes, particularly Aedes aegypti. These mosquitoes are most active during the day, with peak biting times in the early morning and late afternoon. Unlike other mosquito species, Aedes mosquitoes prefer to breed in clean, stagnant water sources found in and around human dwellings, such as flower pots, discarded tires, and water storage containers. The proximity of these breeding sites to human populations contributes to the rapid spread of dengue fever in urban areas.

The transmission of dengue fever can also occur through blood transfusion, organ transplantation, or from an infected mother to her newborn during childbirth. However, these modes of transmission are relatively rare compared to mosquito-borne transmission.

Efforts to control dengue fever primarily focus on reducing mosquito populations and preventing mosquito bites. This includes measures such as eliminating mosquito breeding sites, using insecticides to kill adult mosquitoes, and promoting the use of protective measures like bed nets and insect repellents. Community engagement and education play a crucial role in raising awareness about dengue fever and encouraging individuals to take preventive measures.

The global impact of dengue fever is significant, with an estimated 390 million infections occurring each year. The disease is endemic in more than 100 countries, mainly in Asia, the Pacific, the Americas, Africa, and the Caribbean. Dengue fever poses a substantial burden on healthcare systems, as it can lead to hospitalizations and even death in severe cases. The economic impact of dengue fever is also substantial, with costs associated with medical treatment, vector control efforts, and productivity losses.

In recent years, the incidence of dengue fever has been increasing, partly due to factors such as urbanization, population growth, and climate change. Urbanization creates favorable breeding sites for mosquitoes, while population growth leads to increased human-mosquito contact. Climate change can influence the distribution and abundance of mosquitoes, as well as the transmission dynamics of the dengue virus.

Aedes aegypti mosquitoes are the main carriers of the virus that causes dengue fever. It is characterized by symptoms such as a high fever, a severe headache, joint and muscle pain, and a rash. Dengue fever can progress to more severe forms, such as DHF and DSS, which can be life-threatening.

Efforts to control dengue fever focus on reducing mosquito populations and preventing mosquito bites. The global impact of dengue fever is significant, with millions of infections occurring annually and substantial healthcare and economic burdens. Factors such as urbanization, population growth, and climate change contribute to the rapid spread of dengue fever.

## History and Global Impact of Dengue Fever

Dengue fever, also known as breakbone fever, is a mosquito-borne viral disease that has been a significant public health concern for centuries. This section explores the history of dengue fever and its global impact, shedding light on the magnitude of the problem and the challenges it poses to healthcare systems worldwide.

### Historical Background

The earliest recorded outbreak of dengue fever occurred in China during the Jin Dynasty in the 3rd century AD. The Chinese referred to the disease as "water poison" due to its association with stagnant water sources. Throughout history, dengue fever has been known by various names, including "breakbone fever" in the Caribbean and "dandy fever" in the Americas.

The first documented epidemic of dengue fever in the modern era occurred in 1779–1780 in Asia, Africa, and North America. The disease spread rapidly among British troops stationed in India, leading to thousands of cases and numerous fatalities. Subsequent outbreaks occurred in the 19th century, affecting regions such as Southeast Asia, the Caribbean, and the Americas.

## Global Impact

In recent decades, dengue fever has emerged as a major global health concern. The disease is prevalent in more than 100 countries, primarily in tropical and subtropical regions. The World Health Organization (WHO) estimates that approximately 390 million dengue infections occur annually, with around 96 million cases manifesting clinically. This staggering number highlights the significant burden dengue fever places on healthcare systems worldwide.

Dengue fever has a profound impact on affected individuals, families, and communities. The disease can cause severe flu-like symptoms, including a high fever, a severe headache, joint and muscle pain, and a rash. In some cases, dengue fever can progress to a severe form known as dengue hemorrhagic fever (DHF) or dengue shock syndrome (DSS), which can be life-threatening.

The economic burden of dengue fever is also substantial. The costs associated with medical care, hospitalization, and loss of productivity due to illness can be overwhelming for individuals and communities, particularly in low- and middle-income countries where the disease is most prevalent.

The WHO estimates that dengue fever costs approximately $8.9 billion annually in direct medical costs alone.

## Global Spread and Factors Contributing to Dengue Transmission

The global spread of dengue fever can be attributed to several factors. One key factor is the expansion of the mosquito vectors responsible for transmitting the disease, primarily Aedes aegypti and Aedes albopictus. These mosquitoes thrive in urban environments and have adapted to breed in artificial containers, such as discarded tires, flower pots, and water storage containers. Rapid urbanization, population growth, and inadequate waste management contribute to the proliferation of these mosquito vectors.

Another factor contributing to the global spread of dengue fever is increased international travel and trade. Individuals infected with the virus can unknowingly spread it to new regions, where local mosquito populations can then transmit the disease to susceptible individuals. Climate change and environmental factors can influence mosquito vectors, facilitating dengue fever spread.

The impact of dengue fever is not limited to individual countries or regions. The disease poses a significant threat to global health security. Outbreaks can quickly escalate into epidemics, overwhelming healthcare systems, and straining resources. The interconnectedness of our modern world makes it crucial for countries to collaborate and share information to effectively monitor and control the spread of dengue fever.

Dengue fever has a long and complex history, with its global impact becoming increasingly significant in recent years. The disease affects millions of people annually, causing immense suffering and economic burden. Understanding the historical context and global spread of dengue fever is essential for developing effective prevention and control strategies to mitigate its impact on public health.

## Modes of Transmission and Vector Control

The main methods of transmission for dengue fever are the bites of infected female Aedes mosquitoes, especially Aedes aegypti and Aedes albopictus. These mosquitoes are commonly found in tropical and subtropical regions around the world. Understanding the modes of transmission and implementing effective vector control measures are crucial to preventing and controlling the spread of dengue fever.

### Modes of Transmission

Dengue fever is transmitted in two primary ways: mosquito-borne transmission and vertical transmission.

#### 1. Mosquito-Borne Transmission

Mosquito-borne transmission is the most common mode of dengue fever transmission. When a female

Aedes mosquito bites a person infected with the dengue virus, it becomes infected. After an incubation period of 8 to 10 days, the mosquito becomes capable of transmitting the virus to other individuals. When an infected mosquito bites a healthy person, it injects the virus into the bloodstream, leading to the development of dengue fever.

It is crucial to note that dengue fever is not directly transmitted from person to person. Mosquitoes act as the intermediate vector, transmitting the virus between infected and susceptible individuals. This mode of transmission highlights the significance of controlling mosquito populations to prevent the spread of dengue fever.

## 2. Vertical Transmission

Vertical transmission refers to the transmission of the dengue virus from an infected mother to her child during pregnancy or childbirth. Although vertical transmission is relatively rare, it can occur and result in congenital dengue fever. Infants born to mothers with dengue fever may experience various complications, including low birth weight, preterm birth, and other health issues. Preventing vertical transmission requires effective management and control of dengue fever in pregnant women.

## Vector Control

Vector control plays a crucial role in preventing and controlling the transmission of dengue fever. It involves various strategies and interventions aimed at reducing mosquito populations and interrupting the transmission cycle. Some key vector control measures include:

### 1. Environmental Management

Environmental management focuses on eliminating or reducing mosquito breeding sites. Aedes mosquitoes typically breed in stagnant water sources, such as discarded tires, flower pots, and water storage containers. By promoting proper waste management, regular cleaning of water storage areas, and eliminating standing water, the breeding sites for mosquitoes can be significantly reduced. This approach is particularly effective in urban areas where Aedes mosquitoes thrive in artificial water containers.

### 2. Biological Control

Biological control involves the use of natural enemies of mosquitoes to reduce their populations. One common method is the introduction of larvivorous fish, such as guppies and mosquitofish, into water bodies where Aedes mosquitoes breed. These fish feed on mosquito larvae, thereby reducing the number of adult mosquitoes. Additionally, the use of bacterial larvicides, such as Bacillus thuringiensis israelensis

(Bti), can be effective in controlling mosquito larvae without harming other organisms.

## 3. Chemical Control

Chemical control involves the use of insecticides to kill adult mosquitoes or disrupt their breeding cycle. Indoor residual spraying (IRS) and space spraying are commonly used methods to control adult mosquitoes. IRS involves the application of insecticides on the walls and surfaces of houses, while space spraying involves the use of aerosol insecticides to kill adult mosquitoes in indoor or outdoor spaces. It is important to use insecticides approved for mosquito control and follow proper safety guidelines to minimize environmental and health risks.

## 4. Personal Protection Measures

Personal protection measures are essential in reducing the risk of mosquito bites and dengue fever transmission. These measures include wearing long-sleeved clothing, using mosquito repellents, and sleeping under bed nets. Additionally, community-wide efforts to promote personal protection measures can significantly contribute to reducing the overall mosquito population and preventing dengue fever outbreaks.

## 5. Integrated Vector Management (IVM)

Integrated Vector Management (IVM) is a comprehensive approach that uses multiple vector control strategies to achieve effective and sustainable dengue fever control. IVM involves the integration of environmental management, biological control, chemical control, and personal protection measures. By combining these strategies, IVM aims to target different stages of the mosquito life cycle and reduce mosquito populations more effectively.

Implementing a combination of these vector control measures is crucial to reducing the transmission of dengue fever. It requires collaboration between various stakeholders, including government agencies, healthcare providers, community organizations, and individuals. By adopting a multi-faceted approach, it is possible to mitigate the impact of dengue fever and prevent its rapid spread.

# Chapter 2

# Clinical Manifestations and Diagnosis

## Symptoms and Severity of Dengue Fever

Dengue fever, caused by the dengue virus, is a mosquito-borne disease that affects millions of people worldwide. It is characterized by a wide range of symptoms, ranging from mild to severe. Understanding the symptoms and their severity is crucial for early diagnosis and appropriate management of the disease.

## Mild Symptoms

In many cases, dengue fever presents with mild symptoms that can be mistaken for other common illnesses. The symptoms usually appear 4–7 days after a mosquito bite. The initial signs of dengue fever include a high fever, headache, and muscle and joint pain. These symptoms are often accompanied by a rash, which may appear as small red spots or patches on the skin.

Other mild symptoms of dengue fever may include fatigue, nausea, vomiting, and mild bleeding from the nose or gums. These symptoms can last for about a week and gradually subside without any specific treatment. However, it is important to note that even mild cases of dengue fever can progress to severe forms of the disease.

## Severe Symptoms

Severe dengue, also known as dengue hemorrhagic fever (DHF) or dengue shock syndrome (DSS), is a potentially life-threatening condition. It occurs when the immune response to the dengue virus becomes excessive, leading to increased vascular permeability and abnormal bleeding.

The symptoms of severe dengue may include severe abdominal pain, persistent vomiting, rapid breathing, bleeding gums, blood in vomit or stools, and restlessness. Patients with severe dengue may also experience organ damage, such as liver enlargement or dysfunction and fluid accumulation in the lungs.

One of the most critical complications of severe dengue is dengue shock syndrome, which is characterized by a sudden drop in blood pressure. This can lead to organ failure and even death if not promptly treated. Early recognition of these severe symptoms is crucial for timely medical intervention and management.

## Warning Signs

In addition to the mild and severe symptoms, certain warning signs indicate the progression of dengue fever to a more severe form. These warning signs should not be ignored and require immediate medical attention. Some of the warning signs include:

- Severe abdominal pain or tenderness
- Persistent vomiting
- Bleeding from the nose or gums
- Blood in vomit, stools, or urine
- Restlessness or irritability
- Pale, cold, or clammy skin
- Difficulty breathing
- Fatigue or lethargy

If any of these warning signs are present, it is crucial to seek medical care immediately. Early detection and appropriate management can significantly reduce the risk of complications and improve the chances of recovery.

**Severity Grading**

To assess the severity of dengue fever, healthcare professionals use a grading system based on World Health Organization (WHO) guidelines. This system helps in determining the appropriate level of care and treatment required for each patient.

The severity grading of dengue fever is divided into three categories:

- *Grade I:* **Mild Dengue Fever** - Patients with mild symptoms, such as fever, headache, and muscle, and joint pain, without any signs of bleeding or organ involvement.

- *Grade II:* **Dengue Hemorrhagic Fever (DHF)** - Patients with evidence of bleeding, such as a positive tourniquet test, petechiae, or ecchymosis, along with thrombocytopenia (low platelet count).

- *Grade III:* **Dengue Shock Syndrome (DSS)** - Patients with DHF who develop signs of circulatory failure, such as rapid and weak pulse, narrow pulse pressure, or hypotension.

The severity grading helps healthcare providers determine the appropriate level of care, monitoring, and treatment required for each patient. It also aids in identifying patients who are at a higher risk of developing severe complications.

Dengue fever can present with a wide range of symptoms, varying from mild to severe. Mild cases are often characterized by fever, headache, and muscle, and joint pain, while severe cases can lead to organ damage, abnormal bleeding, and even death. Recognizing the symptoms and their severity is crucial for early diagnosis, appropriate management, and the prevention of complications. If any warning signs or severe symptoms are present, immediate medical attention should be sought to ensure timely intervention and improve patient outcomes.

## Diagnostic Methods for Dengue Fever

Accurate and timely diagnosis of dengue fever is crucial for effective management and control of the disease. Early detection allows for appropriate medical intervention, reducing the risk of severe complications and mortality. In this section, we will explore the various diagnostic methods available for identifying dengue fever.

### Clinical Diagnosis

Clinical diagnosis plays a vital role in the initial identification of dengue fever cases. Healthcare professionals rely on a combination of symptoms, medical history, and physical examination to make a preliminary diagnosis. Common symptoms of dengue fever include high fever, severe headache, joint and muscle pain, rash, and mild bleeding manifestations such as nosebleeds or gum bleeding. However, these symptoms can be similar to those of other viral infections, making clinical diagnosis challenging.

### Laboratory Diagnosis

Laboratory tests are essential for confirming the diagnosis of dengue fever and differentiating it from other similar illnesses. Several diagnostic methods are available, each with its own advantages and limitations. The choice of test depends on the stage of the disease, the availability of resources, and the specific requirements of the healthcare setting.

### 1. Molecular Tests

Molecular tests, such as polymerase chain reaction (PCR), are highly sensitive and specific for detecting the presence of the dengue virus in a patient's blood. PCR can identify the virus even during the early stages of infection when viral levels are low. This method amplifies the viral genetic material, allowing for an accurate diagnosis. However, PCR requires specialized laboratory equipment and trained personnel, making it less accessible in resource-limited settings.

### 2. Serological Tests

Serological tests detect the presence of antibodies produced by the immune system in response to dengue infection. These tests are classified into two types: nonstructural protein (NS1) antigen detection and antibody detection.

NS1 antigen detection tests are rapid and can detect the viral protein within the first few days of infection. These tests are particularly useful for early diagnosis. However, NS1 antigen levels decrease as the infection progresses, limiting their effectiveness in later stages.

Antibody detection tests, such as enzyme-linked immunosorbent assays (ELISA) and rapid diagnostic tests (RDTs), detect the presence of dengue-specific antibodies in the patient's blood. IgM antibodies are typically present during the acute phase of the infection, while IgG antibodies indicate a past infection or immunity.

These tests are widely available, cost-effective, and provide results within a short period of time. However, they may yield false-positive or false-negative results, especially in areas with high rates of cross-reactivity with other flaviviruses.

### 3. Viral Isolation

Viral isolation involves the culture of the dengue virus from a patient's blood sample. This method is time-consuming and requires specialized laboratory facilities. It is primarily used for research purposes and is not commonly employed for routine diagnosis.

### Point-of-Care Tests

Point-of-care tests (POCTs) are rapid diagnostic tests that can be performed at the bedside or in primary healthcare settings. These tests provide quick results, allowing for immediate decision-making and appropriate patient management. POCTs are particularly useful in resource-limited areas where access to laboratory facilities is limited. However, their sensitivity and specificity may vary, and they are not as reliable as laboratory-based tests.

Various POCTs are available, including lateral flow assays and immunochromatographic tests. These tests detect the presence of dengue-specific antigens or antibodies in a patient's blood or serum. While POCTs offer convenience and speed, they may have lower sensitivity compared to laboratory-based tests, leading to potential false-negative results.

Accurate and timely diagnosis of dengue fever is crucial for effective management and control of the disease. A clinical diagnosis provides an initial assessment, but laboratory tests are necessary for confirmation. Molecular tests, such as PCR, are highly sensitive but require specialized equipment and expertise.

Serological tests, including NS1 antigen detection and antibody detection, are widely used and accessible. Viral isolation is primarily used for research purposes. Point-of-care tests offer rapid results but may have lower sensitivity. A combination of these diagnostic methods, along with careful clinical evaluation, can help healthcare professionals accurately diagnose dengue fever and provide appropriate care to patients.

## Differential Diagnosis and Misdiagnosis

Since dengue fever is a virus spread by mosquitoes, it can be difficult to distinguish it from other diseases. The symptoms of dengue fever can often be mistaken for other illnesses, leading to misdiagnosis and delayed treatment. In this section, we will explore the differential diagnosis of dengue fever and the potential pitfalls in diagnosing this disease.

### Differential Diagnosis

There are numerous symptoms associated with dengue fever, which can range in severity from mild to severe. The initial symptoms of dengue fever are similar to those of many other viral infections, such as the flu or common cold. Patients may experience high fever, headache, muscle and joint pain, fatigue, and rash. These nonspecific symptoms make it challenging to differentiate dengue fever from other viral illnesses based solely on clinical presentation.

One of the key differentiating factors of dengue fever is the presence of severe joint and muscle pain, often referred to as "breakbone fever." This symptom, along with the sudden onset of a high fever, can help distinguish dengue fever from other viral infections. However, relying solely on clinical symptoms can lead to misdiagnosis, as other diseases can also cause similar symptoms.

To accurately diagnose dengue fever, healthcare professionals need to consider several factors, including the patient's travel history, exposure to mosquito bites, and the prevalence of dengue fever in the region. Laboratory tests are crucial in confirming the diagnosis and ruling out other diseases. The most commonly used diagnostic test for dengue fever is the detection of viral RNA or antigens in the patient's blood.

## Misdiagnosis

Misdiagnosis of dengue fever can have serious consequences, as delayed or incorrect treatment can lead to complications and even death. Several factors contribute to the misdiagnosis of dengue fever, including the similarity of symptoms to other viral infections, limited access to diagnostic tests in certain regions, and a lack of awareness among healthcare professionals.

One of the common misdiagnoses for dengue fever is influenza, as both diseases share similar symptoms, such as high fever, headaches, and body aches. In regions where dengue fever is endemic, healthcare professionals should consider dengue fever as a differential diagnosis, especially during the peak dengue season. Failure to consider dengue fever as a possibility can result in delayed diagnosis and appropriate treatment.

Another disease that can be mistaken for dengue fever is chikungunya, another mosquito-borne viral infection.

Chikungunya also presents with symptoms such as high fever, joint pain, and rash, making it difficult to differentiate from dengue fever based on clinical presentation alone. Laboratory tests are essential in distinguishing between these two diseases.

In some cases, dengue fever can be misdiagnosed as other viral hemorrhagic fevers, such as Ebola or yellow fever. These diseases can have similar symptoms, including bleeding manifestations, which can lead to confusion in diagnosis. Healthcare professionals must consider the patient's travel history and exposure to specific regions where these diseases are prevalent.

## Challenges in Diagnosis

Diagnosing dengue fever accurately poses several challenges, particularly in resource-limited settings. Access to diagnostic tests, such as polymerase chain reaction (PCR) or enzyme-linked immunosorbent assay (ELISA), may be limited in certain regions, leading to reliance on clinical symptoms alone. This can result in both overdiagnosis and underdiagnosis of dengue fever.

Overdiagnosis occurs when healthcare professionals diagnose dengue fever based solely on clinical symptoms without confirming the presence of the dengue virus. This can lead to unnecessary treatment and increased healthcare costs. On the other hand, underdiagnosis occurs when healthcare professionals fail to consider dengue fever as a possibility, leading to delayed or incorrect treatment.

Improving access to diagnostic tests and increasing awareness among healthcare professionals about the differential diagnosis of dengue fever are crucial steps in reducing misdiagnosis. Rapid diagnostic tests that are affordable, easy to use, and provide quick results can greatly aid in the accurate and timely diagnosis of dengue fever, particularly in resource-limited settings.

The differential diagnosis of dengue fever can be challenging due to the similarity of symptoms with other viral infections. Misdiagnosis can lead to delayed or incorrect treatment, posing a risk to patients. Healthcare professionals need to consider the patient's travel history, exposure to mosquito bites, and the regional prevalence of dengue fever when diagnosing this disease. Access to diagnostic tests and increased awareness among healthcare professionals are essential to reducing misdiagnosis and improving patient outcomes.

# Chapter 3

# Epidemiology and Global Burden

## Epidemiological Trends of Dengue Fever

Dengue fever is a rapidly spreading mosquito-borne viral disease that has become a major public health concern worldwide. In recent years, the epidemiological trends of dengue fever have shown a significant increase in both the number of cases and the geographical spread of the disease.

This section will explore the key epidemiological trends of dengue fever, including the incidence rates, affected populations, and factors contributing to its spread.

## Incidence Rates

The incidence rates of dengue fever have been steadily rising over the past few decades. According to the World Health Organization (WHO), it is estimated that there are around 390 million dengue infections worldwide every year, with approximately 96 million cases manifesting clinically. These numbers highlight the alarming scale of the disease and its impact on global health.

The incidence rates of dengue fever vary across different regions and countries. Southeast Asia, the Western Pacific, and the Americas are the most affected regions, accounting for the majority of dengue cases. In these areas, the incidence rates have been increasing rapidly, with periodic outbreaks occurring every few years.

The reasons for the high incidence rates in these regions can be attributed to various factors, including favorable climatic conditions, urbanization, and inadequate vector control measures.

**Affected Populations**

Dengue fever can affect people of all ages and backgrounds, but certain populations are more vulnerable to the disease. Children, particularly those under the age of 15, are at a higher risk of severe dengue infection. This is partly due to their immature immune systems, which make them more susceptible to the virus.

Additionally, individuals who have previously been infected with one serotype of the dengue virus are at a higher risk of developing severe dengue if they are subsequently infected with a different serotype.

Urban areas with high population densities are also more prone to dengue outbreaks. The presence of stagnant water in urban environments provides breeding grounds for Aedes mosquitoes, the primary vectors of dengue. Moreover, urbanization often leads to inadequate sanitation and waste management, further exacerbating the spread of the disease.

## Factors Contributing to the Spread

Several factors contribute to the rapid spread of dengue fever. Climate change plays a significant role in the expansion of the disease. Rising temperatures and changing rainfall patterns create favorable conditions for Aedes mosquitoes to breed and thrive. As a result, areas that were previously unaffected by dengue are now at risk of outbreaks.

Globalization and increased travel have also contributed to the spread of dengue fever. Infected individuals can unknowingly carry the virus to new areas, where local mosquito populations can then transmit it to others. This has led to the emergence of dengue in regions where it was previously absent or sporadic.

Inadequate vector control measures are another crucial factor in the spread of dengue fever. Aedes mosquitoes are highly adaptive and can breed in small amounts of water found in containers, tires, and other artificial habitats. Insufficient efforts to eliminate these breeding sites and control mosquito populations have allowed the disease to persist and spread.

Furthermore, socioeconomic factors such as poverty and limited access to healthcare contribute to the burden of dengue fever. In resource-limited settings, where healthcare infrastructure is often inadequate, early detection and timely treatment of dengue cases may be challenging. This can lead to higher morbidity and mortality rates in these areas.

The epidemiological trends of dengue fever demonstrate a significant increase in the number of cases and the geographical spread of the disease. The incidence rates are rising globally, with certain regions experiencing periodic outbreaks. Children and urban populations are particularly vulnerable to dengue, and factors such as climate change, globalization, and inadequate vector control measures contribute to its rapid spread. Addressing these epidemiological trends is crucial for effective dengue prevention and control strategies.

## Global Distribution and Burden of Dengue Fever

Dengue fever is a significant global health concern, with its distribution and burden increasing rapidly over the years. This section explores the global prevalence of dengue fever, highlighting the regions most affected and the burden it places on individuals and healthcare systems worldwide.

### Global Prevalence of Dengue Fever

Dengue fever is endemic in over 100 countries, primarily in tropical and subtropical regions of the world. The disease is most prevalent in Southeast Asia, the Western Pacific, and the

Americas. These regions account for the majority of dengue cases reported globally.

Southeast Asia, including countries such as Thailand, Indonesia, and the Philippines, has experienced a high burden of dengue fever for many years. The Western Pacific region, which includes countries like Malaysia, Vietnam, and Fiji, also faces a significant dengue burden. In the Americas, countries such as Brazil, Mexico, and Colombia have reported a substantial number of dengue cases.

Climate, urbanization, and population density are just a few of the variables that affect the distribution of dengue fever. The Aedes mosquitoes, primarily Aedes aegypti and Aedes albopictus, which transmit the dengue virus, thrive in warm and humid environments. As a result, countries with tropical and subtropical climates are more susceptible to dengue outbreaks.

**Burden of Dengue Fever**

Dengue fever imposes a substantial burden on individuals, communities, and healthcare systems worldwide. The disease can cause severe illness, leading to hospitalization and, in some cases, death. The burden of dengue fever is measured in terms of morbidity, mortality, and economic impact.

## Morbidity

Dengue fever is a major cause of morbidity, with millions of cases reported annually. The symptoms of dengue fever can range from mild to severe, with severe cases often leading to dengue hemorrhagic fever (DHF) or dengue shock syndrome (DSS). DHF and DSS are characterized by plasma leakage, organ impairment, and, in severe cases, death.

The burden of dengue fever extends beyond the immediate illness. Even in mild cases, individuals may experience prolonged fatigue and weakness, impacting their daily activities and productivity. Additionally, the psychological impact of dengue fever, including fear and anxiety, can have long-lasting effects on individuals and their families.

## Mortality

While most cases of dengue fever result in full recovery, severe cases can be fatal. According to the World Health Organization (WHO), dengue fever causes an estimated 10,000 deaths annually. The majority of these deaths occur in children, highlighting the vulnerability of younger populations to severe dengue.

Mortality due to dengue fever is often associated with delayed or inadequate medical care. Early detection and appropriate management of severe cases are crucial to reducing the mortality rate. However, in resource-limited settings, access to healthcare facilities and diagnostic tools may be limited, leading to higher mortality rates.

**Economic Impact**

The economic impact of dengue fever is significant, affecting both individuals and healthcare systems. The direct costs of dengue fever include medical expenses, hospitalization, and treatment. Indirect costs, such as lost productivity and income, also contribute to the economic burden.

In countries with high dengue prevalence, the healthcare system faces increased pressure during dengue outbreaks. Hospitals and clinics may become overwhelmed with dengue cases, putting strain on resources and healthcare personnel. The cost of managing dengue outbreaks, including vector control measures and public health campaigns, further adds to the economic burden.

Dengue fever is a global health challenge, with its distribution and burden expanding rapidly. The disease is endemic in numerous countries, primarily in tropical and subtropical regions. Southeast Asia, the Western Pacific, and the Americas bear the highest burden of dengue fever.

The morbidity and mortality associated with dengue fever, particularly in severe cases, highlight the importance of early detection and appropriate medical care. The economic impact of dengue fever further emphasizes the need for effective prevention and control strategies.

## Factors Influencing Dengue Transmission and Outbreaks

It is a complicated disease, with a number of factors influencing its transmission and outbreaks. Understanding these factors is crucial for effective prevention and control strategies. In this section, we will explore the key factors that influence the transmission and outbreaks of dengue fever.

### Environmental Factors

Environmental factors play a significant role in the transmission of dengue fever. The Aedes mosquitoes, primarily Aedes aegypti and Aedes albopictus, which are responsible for transmitting the dengue virus, thrive in warm and humid climates. Therefore, regions with tropical and subtropical climates are more prone to dengue outbreaks.

Rainfall patterns also influence the breeding and survival of Aedes mosquitoes. Long periods of stagnant water after a heavy rain create mosquito breeding grounds. Areas with inadequate sanitation and water management systems are particularly vulnerable to dengue transmission as stagnant water accumulates in containers, discarded tires, and other objects that serve as breeding sites for mosquitoes.

Urbanization and population growth also contribute to the spread of dengue fever. Rapid urbanization often leads to overcrowding, inadequate housing, and poor waste management, creating favorable conditions for mosquito breeding. Additionally, urban areas with a high population density provide a larger pool of potential hosts for the virus, increasing the risk of transmission.

## Socioeconomic Factors

Socioeconomic factors play a crucial role in dengue transmission and outbreaks. Poverty and limited access to healthcare services are significant contributors to the spread of the disease. In impoverished communities, individuals may lack proper housing, sanitation, and access to clean water, creating an environment conducive to mosquito breeding. Moreover, limited access to healthcare facilities may result in delayed diagnosis and treatment, allowing the virus to spread further.

Education and awareness also play a vital role in dengue prevention. Communities with low levels of education and awareness about dengue fever may not understand the importance of vector control measures or may have misconceptions about the disease. This lack of knowledge can hinder effective prevention efforts and contribute to the persistence of dengue transmission.

## Vector Control Measures

The effectiveness of vector control measures significantly influences the transmission and outbreaks of dengue fever. Aedes mosquitoes are known for their adaptability and resilience, making their control challenging. Inadequate vector control measures can lead to the proliferation of mosquitoes and subsequent dengue outbreaks.

Integrated vector management (IVM) is a comprehensive approach that combines various strategies to control mosquito populations. These strategies include environmental management, such as removing stagnant water sources and improving waste management, as well as the use of insecticides and biological control methods. Implementing IVM programs consistently and effectively is crucial for reducing mosquito populations and preventing dengue transmission.

Community participation is essential for the success of vector control measures. Engaging communities in dengue prevention efforts, such as through clean-up campaigns and educational programs, can help raise awareness and promote behavior change. By involving the community, vector control efforts can be more targeted and sustainable, leading to a reduction in dengue transmission.

Understanding these factors and their interactions is essential for developing comprehensive and targeted strategies to control dengue fever. By addressing the environmental, socioeconomic, and vector control aspects, we can mitigate the impact of dengue outbreaks and reduce the burden of this rapidly spreading mosquito-borne disease.

# Chapter 4

# Prevention and Control Strategies

## Vector Control Measures for Dengue Prevention

Vector control plays a crucial role in preventing the transmission of dengue fever. The Aedes mosquito is the main vector of dengue, so taking effective vector control measures is crucial to lowering the risk of dengue outbreaks. This section will discuss various strategies and approaches that can be employed to control the Aedes mosquito population and prevent the spread of dengue.

## Environmental Management

One of the fundamental approaches to vector control is environmental management. This strategy focuses on eliminating or modifying mosquito breeding sites to reduce the population of Aedes mosquitoes. Aedes mosquitoes typically breed in stagnant water sources, such as discarded tires, flower pots, and water storage containers. By removing or properly managing these potential breeding sites, the chances of mosquito proliferation can be significantly reduced.

Regular inspection and cleaning of water storage containers, gutters, and other areas where water can accumulate are essential. Additionally, proper waste management practices, such as disposing of discarded containers and tires, can help eliminate potential breeding grounds for mosquitoes. Implementing these measures not only reduces the risk of dengue transmission but also contributes to overall public health by preventing the spread of other mosquito-borne diseases.

## Biological Control

Biological control methods involve the use of natural enemies or predators to target and control the mosquito population. One effective biological control measure is the introduction of larvivorous fish, such as Gambusia affinis (mosquito fish), into water bodies where Aedes mosquitoes breed. These fish feed on mosquito larvae, thereby reducing the mosquito population.

Another biological control approach is the use of bacteria called Bacillus thuringiensis israelensis (Bti). Bti produces toxins that specifically target mosquito larvae, causing their death. This environmentally friendly method has been successfully used in many dengue-endemic areas to control the Aedes mosquito population.

## Chemical Control

Chemical control measures involve the use of insecticides to kill adult mosquitoes or disrupt their breeding cycle. Insecticides can be applied through various methods, including indoor residual spraying, space spraying, and larviciding.

Indoor residual spraying involves applying insecticides to the walls and surfaces of houses, where mosquitoes rest. This method helps to kill mosquitoes that come into contact with the treated surfaces, reducing their population indoors. Space spraying, also known as fogging, involves the dispersion of insecticides in the form of fine droplets to kill adult mosquitoes in outdoor areas. Larviciding, on the other hand, targets mosquito larvae by applying insecticides directly to their breeding sites.

While chemical control measures can be effective in reducing mosquito populations, it is important to use them judiciously and responsibly. To reduce any potential risks to the environment and human health, trained professionals should choose the appropriate insecticides and apply them correctly.

## Source Reduction

Source reduction is a proactive approach that aims to eliminate or modify mosquito breeding sites to prevent the emergence of mosquito populations. This strategy involves identifying and addressing potential breeding sites in the community, such as stagnant water in discarded containers, blocked drains, and unused swimming pools.

Community involvement is crucial for the success of source reduction efforts. Public awareness campaigns can educate individuals about the importance of eliminating stagnant water sources and maintaining clean surroundings. By actively participating in source reduction activities, communities can significantly contribute to reducing the risk of dengue transmission.

## Integrated Vector Management

Integrated Vector Management (IVM) is a comprehensive approach that combines multiple vector control strategies to achieve effective and sustainable dengue prevention. IVM involves the integration of environmental management, biological control, chemical control, and community engagement strategies.

By combining different control measures, IVM aims to target the mosquito population at various stages of their life cycle and disrupt their breeding and transmission cycles. This approach not only reduces the reliance on a single control method but also increases the overall effectiveness of dengue prevention efforts.

IVM requires collaboration and coordination among various stakeholders, including government agencies, healthcare professionals, community leaders, and the public. By working together, these stakeholders can develop and implement tailored vector control strategies that are suitable for the local context and effectively address the specific challenges posed by dengue transmission.

## Community Engagement and Education for Dengue Prevention

Community engagement and education play a crucial role in preventing the spread of dengue fever. By raising awareness and empowering individuals and communities, we can effectively reduce the transmission of the disease and mitigate its impact. This section will explore the importance of community engagement and education in dengue prevention and provide strategies for implementing effective programs.

### The Role of Community Engagement

Community engagement is a fundamental aspect of dengue prevention, as it involves actively involving individuals, families, and communities in the decision-making process and implementation of preventive measures. By engaging the community, we can foster a sense of ownership and responsibility, leading to sustained efforts in dengue control. Here are some key points regarding the role of community engagement:

- **Empowering individuals:** Community engagement empowers individuals to take charge of their own health and the health of their community. By providing them with knowledge and resources, individuals can make informed decisions and take appropriate actions to prevent dengue transmission.

- **Building trust and cooperation:** Engaging the community helps build trust and cooperation between healthcare providers, local authorities, and community members. This collaboration is essential for the effective implementation of preventive measures and outbreak response.

- **Tailoring interventions:** Community engagement allows for the customization of interventions based on the specific needs and characteristics of the community. By understanding the local context, cultural practices, and social dynamics, interventions can be designed to be more effective and sustainable.

## Strategies for Community Engagement

To effectively engage communities in dengue prevention, it is essential to employ strategies that are inclusive, participatory, and culturally sensitive. Here are some strategies that have proven to be successful:

- **Health education campaigns:** Conducting health education campaigns is an effective way to raise awareness about dengue fever and its prevention. These campaigns can be conducted through various channels, such as community meetings, schools, religious institutions, and mass media. The information provided should be clear, concise, and culturally appropriate, addressing common misconceptions and promoting preventive behaviors.

- **Community mobilization:** Mobilizing the community involves actively involving community members in planning and implementing dengue prevention activities. This can be achieved through the formation of community-based organizations or task forces dedicated to dengue control. These groups can organize clean-up campaigns, distribute educational materials, and monitor mosquito breeding sites in their neighborhoods.
- **Training of community health workers:** Training community health workers (CHWs) is an effective strategy to enhance community engagement. CHWs can be trained to provide accurate information about dengue prevention, identify and report cases, and assist in vector control activities. They can also serve as a bridge between the community and healthcare providers, ensuring timely access to healthcare services.

- **School-based programs:** Schools provide an excellent platform for dengue prevention education. Incorporating dengue prevention into the curriculum can help raise awareness among students and their families. Schools can organize educational activities, such as competitions, plays, and workshops, to engage students and promote preventive behaviors.

- **Social and behavior change communication:** Effective communication strategies are essential for behavior change. Utilizing various communication channels, such as social media, radio, and community gatherings, can help disseminate information about dengue prevention. Messages should be tailored to the target audience, addressing their specific concerns and motivating them to adopt preventive behaviors.

**Overcoming Challenges in Community Engagement**

While community engagement is crucial for dengue prevention, some challenges need to be addressed to ensure its effectiveness. Here are some key challenges and strategies to overcome them:

- **Language and cultural barriers:** Language and cultural differences can hinder effective communication and engagement. To overcome this challenge, it is important to use local languages and culturally appropriate materials. Engaging community leaders and influencers who are respected within the community can also help bridge the gap.

- **Limited resources:** Limited resources can pose a challenge in implementing community engagement programs. To overcome this, partnerships with local organizations, businesses, and government agencies can be established to leverage resources and support. Additionally, seeking funding from international organizations and grants can help sustain community engagement efforts.

- **Sustainability:** Sustaining community engagement efforts over the long term can be challenging. To ensure sustainability, it is important to build capacity within the community by training local volunteers and leaders. Empowering the community to take ownership of the prevention efforts and integrating dengue prevention into existing healthcare systems can also contribute to sustainability.

## Vaccines and Other Preventive Measures

Vaccines and other preventive measures play a crucial role in controlling the spread of dengue fever. While there is currently no specific antiviral treatment for dengue, the development and implementation of effective vaccines can significantly reduce the burden of the disease. In this section, we will explore the progress made in vaccine development as well as other preventive measures that can be employed to combat dengue.

## Vaccine Development

The development of a dengue vaccine has been a long and challenging process. However, significant advancements have been made in recent years, bringing us closer to the goal of having a safe and effective vaccine. Several vaccine candidates have undergone clinical trials, and a few have been licensed for use in certain countries.

The Sanofi Pasteur-developed Dengvaxia vaccine is one of the most promising vaccine candidates. Dengvaxia is a tetravalent vaccine, meaning it protects against all four serotypes of the dengue virus. Clinical trials have shown that Dengvaxia can reduce the incidence of severe dengue and hospitalization in individuals who have previously been infected with dengue. However, its efficacy varies depending on the serostatus of the individual, with higher efficacy observed in those who have had a previous dengue infection.

Another vaccine candidate, TAK-003, developed by Takeda Pharmaceuticals, has shown promising results in clinical trials. TAK-003 is also a tetravalent vaccine and has demonstrated efficacy against all four dengue serotypes. It has shown a reduction in the incidence of symptomatic dengue in individuals aged 4 to 16 years.

While these vaccines show promise, there are still challenges to overcome. Further research is required to determine the length of protection offered by the vaccines as well as their effectiveness across a range of age groups and populations. Additionally, the potential risk of vaccine-induced severe dengue in individuals who have not been previously infected with dengue is a concern that requires careful monitoring.

**Other Preventive Measures**

In addition to vaccines, several other preventive measures can be employed to reduce the transmission of dengue fever. These measures focus on vector control and personal protection.

### Vector Control

Vector control measures aim to reduce the population of Aedes mosquitoes, the primary vectors of dengue. This can be achieved through various methods, including:

- **Environmental management:** Eliminating breeding sites by removing stagnant water and properly disposing of containers that can collect water, such as discarded tires, flower pots, and empty bottles.
- **Biological control:** Introducing natural predators of Aedes mosquitoes, such as

larvivorous fish, to water bodies where mosquitoes breed.

- **Chemical control:** Using insecticides to kill adult mosquitoes and larvicides to target mosquito larvae in water sources.
- **Genetic control:** Implementing innovative strategies such as the release of genetically modified mosquitoes that are unable to transmit the dengue virus.

It is important to note that vector control measures should be implemented as part of an integrated approach, combining multiple strategies to achieve maximum effectiveness.

**Personal Protection**

Individuals can also take steps to protect themselves from mosquito bites and reduce their risk of dengue infection. Some personal protective measures include:

- **Using mosquito repellents:** Apply insect repellents containing DEET, picaridin, or the oil of lemon eucalyptus to exposed skin and clothing.
- **Wearing protective clothing:** Covering exposed skin with long-sleeved shirts, long pants, socks, and shoes, especially during peak mosquito activity times, such as dawn and dusk.

- **Using bed nets:** Sleeping under insecticide-treated bed nets, particularly in areas where Aedes mosquitoes are prevalent.
- **Reducing mosquito exposure:** Avoid outdoor activities in areas with high mosquito populations and ensure the use of screens on windows and doors to prevent mosquitoes from entering living spaces.

By combining these preventive measures with vaccination efforts, it is possible to significantly reduce the transmission and impact of dengue fever.

# Chapter 5

# Future Challenges and Research Directions

## Emerging Issues and Challenges in Dengue Control

Dengue fever continues to pose significant challenges for public health authorities worldwide. Despite efforts to control the disease, there are several emerging issues and challenges that need to be addressed to effectively combat the spread of dengue. This section will discuss some of these emerging issues and challenges in dengue control.

## Climate Change and Urbanization

One of the major emerging issues in dengue control is the impact of climate change and urbanization. As global temperatures rise and urban areas expand, the conditions become more favorable for the proliferation of the Aedes mosquito, the primary vector for dengue transmission. Warmer temperatures and increased rainfall create ideal breeding grounds for mosquitoes, leading to higher transmission rates of the dengue virus.

Urbanization also plays a significant role in the spread of dengue. Rapid urbanization often leads to overcrowding, inadequate sanitation, and poor waste management, which contribute to the proliferation of mosquito breeding sites. Additionally, urban areas often lack proper infrastructure for water storage, leading to the accumulation of stagnant water, an ideal breeding ground for mosquitoes.

To address these challenges, it is crucial to implement effective urban planning strategies that prioritize the prevention and control of mosquito breeding sites. This includes improving sanitation infrastructure, implementing proper waste management systems, and promoting community awareness and participation in dengue prevention efforts.

**Dengue Vaccine Development and Distribution**

The development and distribution of an effective dengue vaccine have been significant challenges in dengue control. While several dengue vaccine candidates have been developed, their efficacy and safety have varied. The complexity of the dengue virus, with four distinct serotypes, poses challenges in developing a vaccine that provides long-lasting protection against all serotypes.

Another challenge is the equitable distribution of the dengue vaccine. Access to vaccines is often limited in low-income countries, where the burden of dengue is highest. The cost of vaccines, along with the need for a multi-dose regimen, poses financial barriers for many countries. Additionally, the logistics of vaccine distribution, including cold chain requirements and reaching remote areas, present further challenges.

To overcome these challenges, there is a need for continued research and development of dengue vaccines that provide broad and long-lasting protection against all serotypes. Efforts should also be made to ensure equitable access to vaccines, particularly in low-income countries where the burden of dengue is highest. This may involve collaborations between governments, international organizations, and pharmaceutical companies to reduce vaccine costs and improve distribution networks.

**Vector Resistance and Insecticide Use**

Vector resistance to insecticides is another emerging issue in dengue control. Over time, mosquitoes have developed resistance to commonly used insecticides, making them less effective in controlling mosquito populations. This resistance is primarily due to the overuse and misuse of insecticides, leading to the selection of resistant mosquito populations.

To address this challenge, it is essential to implement integrated vector management strategies that go beyond relying solely on insecticides. This includes the use of alternative vector control methods such as biological control agents, larvicides, and source reduction. Integrated vector management approaches aim to target multiple stages of the mosquito life cycle and reduce reliance on insecticides, thereby minimizing the development of resistance.

Additionally, there is a need for improved surveillance systems to monitor vector resistance and identify emerging resistance patterns. This information can guide the selection and rotation of insecticides to maximize their effectiveness and minimize the development of resistance.

## Advancements in Dengue Research and Treatment

In recent years, significant advancements have been made in the field of dengue research and treatment. Scientists and medical professionals around the world have been working tirelessly to better understand the virus, develop effective diagnostic tools, and discover new treatment options. These advancements offer hope for the millions of people affected by dengue fever each year.

### Improved Diagnostic Techniques

Accurate and timely diagnosis is crucial for effective management of dengue fever. Traditional diagnostic methods, such as serological tests and viral isolation, have limitations in terms of sensitivity and specificity. However, recent advancements have led to the development of more reliable and efficient diagnostic techniques.

One such advancement is the introduction of molecular diagnostic tests such as polymerase chain reaction (PCR) and loop-mediated isothermal amplification (LAMP). These techniques allow for the detection of dengue virus RNA in patient samples, enabling an early and accurate diagnosis. PCR and LAMP have shown higher sensitivity and specificity compared to traditional methods, making them valuable tools in dengue diagnosis.

Additionally, rapid diagnostic tests (RDTs) have been developed to provide quick and easy detection of dengue virus antigens in patient blood samples. These tests are simple to use and can provide results within a short period of time, allowing for immediate diagnosis and timely initiation of treatment. RDTs have proven to be particularly useful in resource-limited settings where access to laboratory facilities is limited.

**Antiviral Therapies**

Currently, there are no specific antiviral drugs available for the treatment of dengue fever. The management of dengue primarily focuses on supportive care to alleviate symptoms and prevent complications. However, recent advancements in antiviral research have shown promising results in the development of potential therapies for dengue.

One approach being explored is the use of antiviral drugs that target specific stages of the dengue virus life cycle. For example, inhibitors of viral entry, such as small-molecule inhibitors and neutralizing antibodies, have shown potential in preventing viral replication and reducing disease severity. Similarly, drugs targeting viral replication enzymes, such as protease inhibitors and polymerase inhibitors, are being investigated for their efficacy against the dengue virus.

Another area of research is the development of host-targeted therapies. These therapies aim to modulate the host immune response to limit viral replication and reduce the severity of dengue symptoms. Immunomodulatory drugs, such as interferons and immune checkpoint inhibitors, have shown promise in preclinical and clinical studies, although further research is needed to determine their safety and efficacy.

**Vaccine Development**

Vaccination is considered one of the most effective strategies for preventing and controlling infectious diseases. In recent years, significant progress has been made in the development of dengue vaccines. The first dengue vaccine, Dengvaxia, was licensed for use in several countries. However, its use has been limited due to concerns regarding its safety and efficacy.

Efforts are underway to develop safer and more effective dengue vaccines. Several vaccine candidates are currently in various stages of clinical development. These vaccines aim to protect against all four dengue virus serotypes as well as offer long-lasting immunity. Some of the vaccine candidates utilize novel approaches, such as live attenuated vaccines, recombinant protein-based vaccines, and viral vector-based vaccines.

In addition to vaccine development, research is also focused on understanding the immune response to dengue infection. This knowledge is crucial for the development of vaccines that induce a robust and protective immune response. Furthermore, studies are being conducted to determine the optimal vaccine strategies, including the timing and number of vaccine doses, to ensure maximum effectiveness.

## Global Collaboration and Efforts for Dengue Control

Dengue fever is a global health concern that requires collaborative efforts from various stakeholders to effectively control and prevent its spread. As the most rapidly spreading mosquito-borne disease, dengue poses a significant challenge to public health systems worldwide. In this section, we will explore the importance of global collaboration and the various efforts being made to control dengue.

### International Organizations and Partnerships

Addressing the complex nature of dengue requires the involvement of international organizations and partnerships. One such organization is the World Health Organization (WHO), which plays a crucial role in coordinating global efforts to control dengue. The WHO provides technical guidance, supports research, and facilitates the exchange of information among countries affected by dengue.

Additionally, regional partnerships have been established to deal with the particular difficulties that various regions of the world face. For example, the Asian Dengue Vaccination Advocacy (ADVA) group brings together experts from Asian countries to promote the use of dengue vaccines and share best practices in dengue control. These collaborations enable countries to learn from each other's experiences and implement effective strategies tailored to their specific contexts.

**Surveillance and Data Sharing**

Accurate and timely surveillance is essential for monitoring the spread of dengue and identifying areas at risk of outbreaks. Global collaboration plays a crucial role in enhancing surveillance systems and promoting data sharing among countries. Through initiatives like the Global Dengue Observatory (GDO), countries can share epidemiological data, research findings, and best practices in dengue control.

The GDO, established by the WHO, serves as a platform for countries to access and contribute to a global database on dengue. This database enables researchers and policymakers to analyze trends, identify high-risk areas, and develop targeted interventions. By sharing data and collaborating on surveillance efforts, countries can collectively strengthen their ability to detect and respond to dengue outbreaks.

## Research and Innovation

Global collaboration is vital for advancing research and innovation in dengue control. Researchers from different countries and institutions work together to develop new diagnostic tools, treatment strategies, and preventive measures. Collaborative research projects allow for the pooling of resources, expertise, and data, leading to more robust scientific findings.

One example of global collaboration in dengue research is the Pediatric Dengue Vaccine Initiative (PDVI). PDVI brings together researchers, policymakers, and funders to accelerate the development and introduction of dengue vaccines specifically for children. By pooling resources and expertise, PDVI aims to address the unique challenges associated with dengue in pediatric populations.

Furthermore, international collaborations facilitate the sharing of research findings and knowledge dissemination. Scientific conferences, workshops, and publications provide platforms for researchers to present their work, exchange ideas, and foster collaborations. This collective effort accelerates the progress of dengue research and brings us closer to effective control and prevention strategies.

## Capacity Building and Training

Global collaboration in dengue control extends beyond research and includes capacity-building and training initiatives. Developing countries often face resource constraints and limited expertise in dealing with dengue outbreaks. Collaborative efforts aim to address these gaps by providing training programs, technical assistance, and capacity-building workshops.

The WHO, in collaboration with partner organizations, conducts training programs on dengue prevention and control for healthcare professionals, vector control personnel, and policymakers. These programs equip participants with the necessary knowledge and skills to effectively manage dengue outbreaks, implement vector control measures, and educate communities.

Additionally, partnerships between academic institutions and public health agencies facilitate the exchange of expertise and knowledge transfer. Through these collaborations, researchers and practitioners from different countries can learn from each other's experiences and develop innovative approaches to dengue control.

## Advocacy and Resource Mobilization

Global collaboration plays a crucial role in advocating for increased political commitment and resource mobilization for dengue control. International organizations, governments, and civil society groups work together to raise awareness about the impact of dengue and the need for sustained investments in prevention and control measures.

Advocacy efforts focus on highlighting the burden of dengue, its economic impact, and the potential benefits of investing in prevention. By mobilizing political will and securing financial resources, global collaborations contribute to the implementation of comprehensive dengue control programs.

# Conclusion

As we have seen, the global spread of dengue represents one of the most serious infectious disease threats facing humanity today. Over the last half-century, dengue has expanded inexorably despite our best efforts, a persistent and complex problem exacerbated by rapid urbanization, climate change, globalization, and inadequate control measures. With over 3 billion people at risk worldwide, no vaccine, and no specific treatments, the potential for recurrent large-scale epidemics is alarming.

Yet this book has also highlighted much progress in dengue research and multiple innovative approaches underway. New vector control technologies, improved surveillance and prediction models, novel mosquito modification strategies, diagnostic advancements, and progress toward an effective multivalent vaccine all offer hope. With strong political commitment, targeted research funding, and evidence-based implementation of integrated prevention programs, the trajectory of the dengue pandemic can be altered.

But there is no single magic bullet. As this book has shown, battling dengue requires a multifaceted arsenal deployed strategically and consistently over the long term. Surveillance, vector control, vaccine implementation, clinical management, public education, and rapid response to outbreaks—each component is critical and must be supported simultaneously. Partnerships between governments, NGOs, academia, industry, and affected communities are also key to maximizing impact.

While much work remains, the outlook is not bleak. We possess the scientific understanding and tools needed to mitigate dengue's toll if applied appropriately in a coordinated global effort. With diligence and continued progress, we can envisage a future where dengue no longer poses an overwhelming burden.

It will require sustained commitment, resources, and the right policies guided by evidence. But by working relentlessly as a united front, we can contain and ultimately reverse the trajectory of the dengue pandemic. The health and prosperity of future generations depend on it.